16 Common Smoking Rationalizations Recognized,
Analyzed And Ultimate Destroyed.

by Andreas Michaelides

16 Common Smoking Rationalizations Recognized, Analyzed And Ultimate Destroyed. Print Version

ISBN: 978-9963-2285-8-4
Cyprus Library.
www.cypruslibrary.gov.cy

Table of Contents

About the Author

Andreas was born in Athens, the city that gave birth to Democracy, in Greece, the country that taught to the world how to live, think, and have fun. He grew up in the beautiful island of Cyprus.

With both of his parents bibliophiles (and his father a high school teacher), Andreas grew up with a love and appreciation for literature. In addition to the books he borrowed from the school library, a stack of encyclopedias taught him about the world. A history lover from age 13, he devoured the memoirs of Winston Churchill and Charles de Gaul, and by age 17, he had read all of Julius Vern's books.

After serving his country for 26 months immediately after finishing high school, Andreas studied in Patra, Greece to become a computer engineer. With his Master of Computer Engineering and Informatics, he began working in the Informatics Department of the local university hospital, and started reading again with a vengeance.

In 2004, Andreas authored his first book, a historical novel that has not yet seen the light of publication. Leaving it unpublished made him feel like a failure, but a lot has changed since then. Eleven years later, he has successfully quit smoking and has been smoke-free for the past six years. He has also started running again and managed to lose 26 kg (57 lbs).

Andreas has run three marathons, as well as many half-marathons and other shorter races. His love for running is what renewed him and actually saved his life.

Multiple medical problems pushed Andreas to research and experiment with a plant-based diet; since 2013 he is following a whole plant based diet.

In addition to running, Andreas enjoys hiking, cycling, playing basketball, camping, photography, and going out with friends and family and having a good time.

Prologue

Warning about length (wink). This story is going to be long, really long, because there is no other way around it. There are no miracles and quick fixes as far as smoking is concerned; you need to learn the truth and the truth is always hiding behind facts, waiting for someone to discover it. The truth is hard evidence and not cheap, short one line sentences like smoking is wrong for you, or smoking kills. They are true but the smoker's mind, like I was eight years ago, doesn't click with messages like that. If you are a smoker, and you have a genuine interest in quitting, read this story from top to bottom.

From 1993 until 2009, I was a cigarette smoker. It started with one cigarette in 1993 and just before I quit, I was smoking 40 cigs a day! And when a student in Greece, I was smoking easily four packs a day!. The only time I wasn't smoking was when I was sleeping, and I was asleep in a room where I smoked the rest of the day. You could see the ceiling had a yellowish color; that's the color nicotine becomes when oxidizes. I am telling you these things so you understand that if I managed to quit, you could stop, too. This article is part of a series with smoking as its central theme. I have some others on my blog; my latest was How to Quit Smoking Forever, where I briefly touch on the method someone must use to have a high rate of success of stopping. It was the way I used to quit smoking, and this year, in May 2016, I will be smoke-free for seven years. I mention in my Smoking chapter of my first book, an autobiography basically, every time a year goes by with not even a puff, it's a cause for celebration because seven years ago, I took my life back; I escaped the prison called Nicotine Addiction. Do not kid yourself, my fellow readers, and especially those who smoke, I was a junkie, I was a drug addict, and my drug was nicotine. The fact that is legal to purchase freely anywhere doesn't make it any less of a drug and me back then and you today a drug addict.

If you grasp this idea of what you are and position yourself as you exist in society, you will make the connections and decide to get rid of your addiction.

Smoking is just one way of being a prisoner of nicotine; there are other ways a person can continue to be in this highly addictive state and not smoke cigarettes. You have chewing tobacco, snuff (very popular in Sweden), you have nicotine chewing gum and nicotine patches. Don't kid yourself, these two are not cures from smoking, they are just another way to keep your mind dull and numb to the dopamine releases nicotine creates. It gives a sense of relief and pleasure, when, in reality, you just satisfy a technical and unnecessary addiction that you set up with your first puff years ago.

In this story, I want to recognize, analyze, and ultimately destroy and kick right out of your head all these rationalizations people who smoke use as an excuse so not to stop smoking.. Rationalizations that I also was bringing as arguments when confronted with the truth by other non-smokers.

There are as many rationalizations about not quitting smoking as the number of smokers out there. Millions. Unfortunately, millions die from cancer and other smoking-related illnesses but even more unfortunate is that those millions are replaced daily by new nicotine addicts. Most of them kids and teenagers, young people, the future of our planet, drugged and giving away their lives.

So I chose 16 of them, and I picked 16 of them because that's how many years I was an ignorant, selfish drug addict with no regard to what was happening around me. The only thing in my mind was to satisfy an addiction, which I created myself, no one else, to meet a false way of life that nicotine imposed on me and finally to satisfy my urges with no regard to the environment around me.

So my fellow people, non-smokers, ex-smokers, and current smokers, let's begin the catharsis, let's learn a few useful truths of what smoking is, what nicotine is, and arm ourselves with some solid truthful, factual arguments to use. The non-smokers and ex-smokers can use them when they talk with other smokers and for the smokers to help them come to that realization point that you are a drug addict, and you need to recover to your previous nicotine free state, because trust me, that state is where you will find your true self.

My name is Andreas Michaelides, and I am a recovering drug addict. My drug was nicotine. Never take another puff in your life, smoke-free and free to live your life.

Rationalization Number One: Just one more won't kill me, or I only did it just once.

Thoughts in smokers' heads are following, I made these rationalizations numerous times myself before I was liberated from the nicotine trap. Tell me if they sound familiar.

• I quit smoking for two months now, I am not addicted anymore, just one cigarette with my friends on Friday night to celebrate won't do any harm.

• It's three years now since I last smoked, I don't think smoking once in a full moon when I watch soccer with my buddies will do something to me.

• I quit seven years ago, but all my girlfriends smoke when we go for drinks, I don't think one little puff now and then just to fit in will make me go back to smoking.

Sound familiar? If it does, and you quit smoking a while ago, it doesn't matter if it's one month or 10 years, UNDERSTAND this, sorry about the caps, but you need to GET IT. One puff and you are back to square one, forget all the years, months, or days that you did not smoke, forget about the withdrawal symptoms you had to endure to reach your drug-free state, they were just annulled. Yes, I am *serious*, you just became a nicotine addict again! Nicotine's addictive properties are that powerful; it only takes one puff for your dopamine receptor pathways in your brain to get saturated by nicotine again!

That's why is so dangerous, that's why we must be extra careful not to allow our kids to take even one puff, that's it, finito, they are hooked!

John R. Polito, in his book, *Freedom from Nicotine – The Journey Home*, a book that every human being on this planet should read, all of us, non-smokers, ex-smokers, smokers, future smokers, all of us, talks about the **Law of Addiction**. This law is so important that an entire chapter in his book is devoted to it.

In a nutshell, this law says that, and I quote, ***"Administration of a drug to an addict will cause re-establishment of chemical dependence upon the addictive substance."***

You cannot escape the Law of Addiction, it is like you being on the edge of a cliff and you are arguing with yourself that if I take a step, I won't fall and kill myself. It's like claiming that the *law* of gravity doesn't apply to you somehow.

Contemplating taking even a little puff from a burning cigarette is like taking a step into the void and thinking you won't fall. Well, you can't, it is a law; you just can't *ignore* a law.

Well, you can ignore it, of course, but you end up being a pitiful drug addict who will spend all their hard earned money, precious time, destroy all their social ties and drive themselves literally to the grave by smoking to satisfy his or her addiction!

I am closing with this: Years ago, I had an incident, and I remember it now when researching for this article and a book I am planning to publish shortly about smoking.

It was June of 2009, I had quit smoking two months before, and I did something dumb. See back then, I knew nicotine was in the cigarette but never knew its addictive powers. I viewed smoking as a bad habit, a nasty habit, and not as an addiction. I only wish I knew back then what I know now, about the law of addiction.

If I knew the depths of my substance abuse and that I was a *drug* addict, that it only takes one puff to return to square one, I would never have smoked a puff from a cigarette my cousin gave me two months after I stopped. In my mind, I had a bad habit that's what I thought in my stupid, ignorant head I took that puff to see if I managed to break free!

I did not smoke another cigarette since then, and that's the honest truth, I was lucky I did not relapse. Maybe I had more strength in me than I thought, maybe the fact that as soon as the cigarette was lit, I felt sick to my stomach and that very tiny puff was so disgusting to my mouth, it kept me away for good.

But next year, I am not going to celebrate my escape from nicotine in May because knowing what I know now, I became an addict again even for the briefest of moments in June. I will celebrate my eight years as a recovering drug addict and away from the drug that kept me in the dark for so many years, nicotine, in June.

Lesson Number 1: Smoking is not a habit, is one of the many ways to deliver Nicotine into your body. Nicotine is a potent addictive agent, and it only takes *one puff* to get hooked. A habit takes three to four weeks for someone to do a task every day, smoking is *not a habit*.

Rationalization Number Two: Smoking helps me relax from stress and anxieties of life.

I am still laughing, not at you, but at my idiotic behavior all the years I was a smoker, a drug addict. This rationalization was one of my most often used, because in my mind, when I was feeling stressed or I was anxious for something, I would grab a cig, put it in my mouth, light it with my zippo, and inhale a long, intense puff down into my lungs; oh, my poor lungs. After that, a sense of tranquility and relaxation occurred. Thus, smoking must have relaxed me when I was stressed or anxious, right? NO, DEAD NO! Sorry about the caps again.

Let's not forget for a moment that I was a drug addict, and I had a drug circulating in my body, bloodstream, and brain, like many of you have in your body, brain, and blood now.

Nicotine doesn't stay there forever, it leaves the body; the body is not stupid, it's a toxin, our sick body is using any means possible to get rid of the poison, but we make sure to refuel it with every puff we take.

Let me give you a few numbers about nicotine and what it does to our body, and then you decide if nicotine, which is what you receive while *smoking*, helps in relaxing you or helps you deal with stress or anxiety. Let's go.

I am going to borrow some information from the smoking chapter from my first book, *Thirsty for Health*.

I am quoting the book,

"Nicotine, a Deadly Poison

You can find nicotine in the tobacco plant, and it has a natural protection from being eaten by insects. Its widespread use as an insecticide for crops is the main culprit for killing honey bees. A toxin, drop for drop, nicotine has proven to be as lethal as strychnine and, in studies performed on animals, is now three times deadlier than arsenic.

Some Nasty Info about Nicotine

Nicotine is highly addictive. The ingestion of nicotine results in a discharge of epinephrine from the adrenal cortex, causing a sudden release of glucose. Stimulation is followed by depression and fatigue, leading the abuser to seek more nicotine.

Nicotine is a highly toxic chemical. In rats, a dose of 50 mg per kg is lethal; in mice, the median lethal dose is around 3 mg per kg; and in humans, the median lethal dose is 0.5 to 1.0 mg/kg (or around 40 to 60 mg in an average human).

This little lethal dose makes nicotine more toxic than many other compounds, even including alkaloids such as cocaine, which has a median lethal dose of 95.1 mg per kg in mice.

As nicotine can be absorbed into the bloodstream quickly through the skin, if an extremely high concentration of nicotine is spilled on the skin, this can lead to toxicity and death."

Now, mind you, I wrote the book after quitting smoking and still I didn't quite grasp the fact that I was a drug addict. I was in the fog of that smoking is a nasty habit. It's this article, research, and the three books I read about smoking that woke me up and shook me to my core. I wish I had the knowledge I have now back then. I am sure it wouldn't have taken four failed attempts to quit, and the one that was successful would be much much easier because I like logic and hard evidence.

I knew that nicotine is poison, I knew it's addictive, but it didn't click that I was a drug addict. I know it's weird and stupid, I suppose I was in denial. The reason I didn't make the association between nicotine and addiction was that I lacked an integral piece of information. This piece of information is the physiological effects stress and anxiety has on your body.

It goes like this, when we are stressed or anxious about something, our urine becomes acidic. You know chemistry, pH under 7 is acidic, above 7 is alkaline. Now the body is not stupid, it cannot have an acidic urine, it's not good for you so what does it do exactly?

Well, if you are a non-smoker, it will take dietary calcium, about 90%, the other 10% it takes from our bones, that's why is so important to have an alkaline diet. Eating lots of fruit and vegetables counteracts the acidity with calcium, which has an alkaline effect, and voila, our urine is back to alkaline, which is good to have.

When you are a smoker, and you are stressed or anxious, your body takes nicotine from your blood and drives it into your urine to make it alkaline, because nicotine is an alkaloid!

Did you get it? Let me repeat so it sticks in your brain. When you stress, or you are anxious, the body removes the nicotine from your bloodstream and uses it to make your urine more alkaline.

What happens when nicotine leaves your bloodstream? Withdrawal symptoms start to appear, what does a smoker do when they start to have withdrawal symptoms? Yes, you got it, he or she smokes to replace the lost nicotine the body had to use to make our urine more alkaline.

The second is that nicotine makes your heart beat 17.5 times faster per minute. I know that when someone is relaxed, he or she is in that beautifully relaxed state when our heart is beating in a slow and stable rhythm. That's relaxing.

When you are sitting down, and your heart is beating 17.5 times more per minute without doing any form of exercise or anything else that would justify the raise of your heart to that level, then I am sorry to say, that's not relaxing.

When I was a smoker, my heart rate was 85 beats per minute and my systolic blood pressure was 13.5. Now after seven years of smoke-free and nicotine free, my heart rate is 50 beats per minute! I know, but that's because I run marathons as a hobby now! And my systolic blood pressure is 11!

The stimulant effect of nicotine clearly shows that it makes your heart goes faster, and that, my friends, is not relaxing. When you are relaxed, you have a relaxed heart rate and not a train that lost control.

The bottom line is when you are stressing, your body loses octane fast, withdrawal symptoms kick in, and you feel the urge to smoke to replenish your nicotine levels into your blood.

When you do that, you are feeding and satisfying your addiction but because you are stressing at the same time, in your head, the pleasure and euphoria you feel translates as a relaxation from your stress. In reality, you are only feeding your nicotine addiction, replenishing nicotine loss as a result of stress and at the same time, physiologically, you are adding more stress to your body by increasing your heart rate by 17.5 per minute.

You need to understand that smoking and nicotine addiction remove your ability to cope with stressful situations. Stress is not a bad thing when you can manage it.

Stress is a way of our body motivating us to do something so we will achieve tasks that need to be doing. A few examples of productive stress are:

Working long hours to complete a critical project

Taking care of family matters that are more urgent than others

A marathoner needing to do a specific amount of exercise

All of these are stressful at times but necessary to achieve our goal. After we reach our goal, the body rewards us with a dose of dopamine, the happy chemical as many call it. The mechanism of dopamine is very complex and this is a crude oversimplification but let's work with it for the moment.

You feel stress, you do something, and you relieve the stress, achieving your goal at the same time, and your body rewards you with beautiful, happy substances. That's a healthy attitude, one that smokers cannot do.

The reason is when a smoker is stressed, instead of thinking how to construct a plan on how to overcome and solve this stressful situation, it does something opposite, it does nothing! And the reason it does nothing is that stress is stealing away his "precious" nicotine from his body. So what do you think a drug addict will do first? Satisfy his/her addiction or confront the situation that stresses him/her out?

Is it pretty obvious, right? He/she is going light a cigarette. Do you know how dangerous this is? Imagine being in a life or death situation and you are traveling with a smoker, how do you think a smoker will react to the stress of an event like that? He will either freeze or light a cigarette, oblivious of the gravity of the situation because after all, he or she is a drug addict just like any other addict. Heroin, cocaine, meth, and so on.

Trust me, I've been there.

Let me tell you a personal experience that shows how a smoker will react in stressful situations. It was night around 10 p.m. I was coming back from one of my night computer classes, I was an IT teacher for five years. I was hungry, I was up at five a.m., and the only thing I ate was a cruller hours ago. So you can imagine the only thing I wanted to do was go home, eat, take a shower, and sleep.

5 minutes before I arrive home, I hit a hole in the road and rips my left front tire of my Golf station wagon to pieces. I manage to control the car and park it safely on the left side of the road. I almost lost control of the car because, guess why? Because I was smoking! But this is not my point.

I extinguish the cig in my car ashtray and get out to see how big of damage I had. I check the tire and realize that it's destroyed.

Now, what do you think was my next move? I was hungry, sleepless, tired from working all day, all these three are stressors enough, right? I needed to change a tire in the middle of nowhere in the dark, something that will take me at least 45 minutes, thus making my arrival home to food, sleep, and rest past midnight, and I needed to wake up at five a.m. the next day, making that a 4-hour sleep!

What do you think all those stressful events I just told you and played in my head would do to my actions?

Before you answer that, let me ask you this.

What would a non-smoker will do? Well, he will open the back door of this car, find his jack and his tools to change the tire, his emergency lights to signal to the other drivers that he is in danger, and then start the procedure to changing his tire so he can get home faster.

What did I DO? I LIGHT A CIGARETE!

I wasted another 5 to 7 minutes smoking because I thought I was dealing with the stressful situation but in reality, I was just feeling the absence of nicotine which occurred from my stress and anxiety. Also, I put myself in danger by not situating the emergency signals in the road, risking being hit by oncoming traffic.

Now after all this information do you honestly believe that smoking relieves stress and anxiety?

Lesson Number 2: Smoking does not reduce stress or anxiety, smoking is replenishing nicotine into your bloodstream that was lost because of stress and anxiety. It's a vicious cycle. The relaxation feelings you have when you smoke when stressed is nothing but the refueling of nicotine, satisfying your withdrawal symptoms like a real drug addict you are.

Rationalization Number Three: Smoking helps me go through hard times; it's my friend.

It is a powerful rationalization because I used it in the past to justify my nicotine addiction to others but also most importantly, and at the same time, terrible for my mental health, I used it as an argument to convince myself.

This rationalization was the one that kept me smoking when I was a student, and I was alone in my little apartment, especially during the winter when it was raining hard outside and nowhere else to go. Smoking was my friend, it did keep me company while I was having my coffee after I ate. It was sweet of it to keep me company while I was watching a movie, it was always there for me, never let me down.

You smokers out there, you know what I mean, you feel me, right? Well, _wrong_, sorry to burst this bubble, but smoking is not your friend, your buddy, your companion. Friends don't hang around with you all the time even when you go to the toilet! Right, do they? Well, you must have some weird friends if they do that.

Friends talk to us when we are down and when we are happy, when did smoking or its twin sister, nicotine, ever speak to you? The answer is never. Do you know how stupid I feel right now that I had to personify a chemical and then had the stupidity to call it a friend?

Wake up, the evil twin siblings (smoking tobacco and nicotine) are not your friend! They are exactly the opposite of that, they are selfish and always conspire to kill you.

A friend will never give you poisons, they will never do anything that will bring your health in danger; friends love you and want what is best for you.

Tell me what smoking or nicotine is doing for your well-being if they are your friends? Tell me one good thing that tobacco use and nicotine does for you to justify your argument that they are your friends, your buddies, your comfort on sad, rainy days?

Well, I tell you. ZILCH, a big NOTHING. On the contrary, they drug you and poison you every day, 3 to 4 thousand chemicals blacken your lungs with every cig, slowly and methodically killing your only way to get fresh air into your body; your little buddies are gradually and intentionally suffocating you to death.

Sure, I can talk through a hole in the base of my throat, why do I have to speak through my mouth?

Friends do not kill their friends.

They don't let you do vigorous tasks like cycling, running, swimming, making love to your wife, for goodness sake, and playing with your kids.

And if that is not enough, to make sure they finish the job, they put around 60 to 80 chemicals in your body that are scientifically proven to cause *cancer*! This includes lung cancer and esophageal cancer. Hey, you have two lungs, right, you can lose one to your buddy the cigarette, I mean, what are friends for?

Before it gives you all the serious diseases and illness, it bothers you on a daily basis with colds and flu and aching and all sorts of other minor but annoying little discomforts because it brings down your immune system, exposing you to a variety or illness and disasters. Is that what a friend would do?

Sure, I can talk through a hole in the base of my throat, why do I have to speak through my mouth?

Friends do not kill their friends.

Do you see what are you doing? You are bringing a nasty habit (the mechanical act of smoking) and a chemical (nicotine) into life in your mind. You gave them anthropomorphic substance, and you are having a dialogue in your head! Like they are human beings. WELL, THEY ARE NOT. WAKE UP!

It's a dirty, nasty habit that delivers a hugely addictive chemical into your brain, suffocating and squeezing the life out of you steadily, gradually, and methodically. It's doing it because you think nicotine is your friend. *No*, nicotine is an addiction you created yourself, it's a chemical, for goodness sake. It cannot feel; it cannot talk, eat, smell, hear, hug you, comfort you, or relax you. Don't use that excuse anymore. I explained in the previous rationalization that smoking does not relax you.

It's like a rock. A rock is a rock, it cannot express any true abilities and nicotine is the same, it's an odorless, colorless, tasteless chemical.

It's not your friend! Stop personifying it. See it for what is, an addictive chemical, nothing more, nothing less.

Lesson Number 3: Smoking and nicotine are *not* your friends. They are 1.) a nasty, dirty method of delivering a 2.) highly addictive chemical into your system. Stop calling them your friends, they are not, hang out with your real friends and stop anthropomorphizing chemicals and get your butt out of the house and into the real world. Socialize and find real friends, not made-up friends in your head. Honestly, now you are not 5 years old anymore to have imaginary friends.

Rationalization Number Four: I don't know about everyone else, I am not like the others, I love smoking. People just don't get how much I like it.

Yep, used that lame excuse myself numerous times when I was under the influence of nicotine, a very addictive chemical. But it is not as hard as you think to break through; I will tell more in another article.

Many people, including me, of course, are ignorant; I may know a great deal on one subject but be completely ignorant on another topic either because I don't care to learn or because the information is not available.

Of course, a drug addict will say that he likes, or loves, smoking or smoking is his/her friend. He is drugged and doesn't know what the hell is talking about. When I was a smoker, my brain was captured and conquered by nicotine. The only thing I was making sure to do was to feed my addiction so I won't feel or a sense or even allow myself to go near withdrawal symptoms, because it's bad. That's what they say to people, that withdrawal symptoms are bad. Excuse my language but that's bullshit. Yes, they are bad, but they are not impossible to overcome.

What exactly does someone like or love about smoking? What? Let's see the beautiful side first. This is for the ladies.

Skin ages faster, wrinkles form faster, your hair smells like you just got out a chimney, your mouth smells like a barbecue and not in a good way, your teeth and fingers become yellow because nicotine, when oxidized with air, turns yellow. Your clothes stink of smoke.

You think someone would love or like to be around you if you are a stinky, wrinkled person with bad mouth odor? Do you? I don't believe so. God, I only imagine what other people were thinking every time I was opening my mouth and talking to them, and that smoke stench was coming out of my mouth and towards their nostrils, opening them and making them puke, but they were polite enough not to say anything. A lot of them will turn away to gasp for air, others will cover their nose to block the nasty odors. I remember now, and I understand why they were doing them.

Others, though, were more direct and honest with me. They would shake their hand in front of their nose, trying to remove the smoke odor from their face and tell me," Oh, my God, you stink !How many cigarettes did you smoke today?", and the funny thing would be that it could be none, the stench was there anyway!

What else do you like about smoking or love about it? It gives you cancer. Do you need any other hard facts for you to reevaluate your rationalization that smoking is not something that you love doing?

You are a drug addict, and that's why you are saying and doing what you are saying and doing.

Let's analyze it a little bit here. I learned how to analyze when I went to university, and one of the first things you need to do before you even write a computer program is to analyze it. If something doesn't work or doesn't have a logical sequence, then you redesign it, so it makes sense. So basically, you have false reasoning and correct logic, you have 0 and 1.

Let's apply this thinking to my cooking.

I like eating kidney beans (red beans). I am cooking them right now as I am writing this lines.

I like eating them because they are good for me, they have fiber, lots of iron I need because I am Vegan, vitamins, phytonutrients, and so on. So I like eating kidney beans because I eat them often.

In the same way, let's see how I will analyze and criticize myself when I was a smoker:

I do things that I like.

I smoke four packs of cigarettes a day.

The conclusion I must like smoking, right? No ,*wrong.*

That's a junkie's thinking; the nicotine doesn't let you see that you are in error.

The right analysis made by a non-smoker, a nondrug addict will be this:

I do things that I like.

I smoke a lot of cigs a day.

Cigarettes kill me every day with their tar and their nicotine.

I am a drug addict who kills him/herself with every puff.

I now know that nicotine is highly addictive.

I tried to quit and failed.

So, I must be a drug addict.

Now this is the analysis and the thinking flow of someone who is waking up from the fog of considering that smoking is something they like to do.

Another thing about saying that you like smoking, what do you like exactly? I am asking again. The morning cough or continuous cough, the sputum that you spit, the dry throat? What, exactly?

It must be the subtle sensations you feel when you replenish your depleted nicotine blood storage. Then, yes, that must be it. There is nothing else to argue that makes you love or like smoking.

When you love or like something, you love it for all it is, not being selective and say I love it for that only. That's drug addict behavior, but then again, that's what you are. That's what I was. You can lose this addiction, and one of the first steps is to recognize the fact the you don't love or like smoking, you're addicted to nicotine and that's why you think you like the act of smoking.

Lesson Number 4: You don't like or love tobacco use. How can you love or like something that kills you little by little every day? You are a drug addict. Admit it, acknowledge it, and start the catharsis procedure now. You love and like things that are good for you. Nicotine is not okay for you, it kills your brain by literally deleting your memory. One puff and hey, what's my name? Another puff there and hey, you forgot your anniversary.

Rationalization Number Five: I am not like the others, I am not that addicted. I can control it. I only smoke a couple of cigs a month and maybe a few on particular occasions, you know, as a treat.

I am a little bit addicted, or I have it under control are just little excuses we tell ourselves to justify and hide our addiction. If it's little addicted then why don't you quit? I mean, it's little, so it must be easier to stop, right? Why don't you just do that? Also, I am in control. The reality is that you are under the control of nicotine. If you are in control, then, again, why don't you stop at once? It's so easy, you are in control, right?

That's what I used to say to myself when I first started smoking the first couple of years. I knew smoking was bad for me, but I had this excuse and rationalization in my head all the time: I am not addicted, it's just a nasty habit. I can stop whenever I want, easily, no hassles, no drama. I realized how wrong I was when five years of smoking and a week before my final exams, I made a decision to quit smoking. I realized how addicted I was to tobacco use and how hard it was to stop. Not so hard concerning my mental state, it was strong, but it was my physiological condition that made me cry like a baby for days before I started smoking again. I describe the attempt in my book, *Thirsty for Health* and also in an article in my blog (put the link here)

There is no little or a lot addicted to smoking, either you are, or you are not. There are no gray areas here.

You are a drug addict, whether you're smoking four packs a day, like I did at some point, or smoking a couple of cigs every month. We are both adults and the ones who say they are in control are the people who don't know their limits. I knew my limit was four packs a day; I know it's sad, and I am so glad I am not filling my lungs with tar anymore and killing my brain cells with nicotine anymore. It doesn't matter if you smoke 80 cigs a day or 5 cigs a day, the chances of a cell turning cancerous is the same.

Lesson Number 5: The bottom line is, whether you smoke one cig a day or 20 or 40 or more, you are a nicotine addict. You lost the ability to think for yourself because you have a drug in your bloodstream that makes you think and acts not like yourself.

Rationalization Number Six: I like smoking because of the excellent flavor/taste they have.

Really? You like smoking because of the flavor/taste. Hmm, interesting, considering that the smoke from the cigarette feels awful, and the flavor is artificially enhanced and added by the tobacco companies to hook you even more into your nicotine addiction.

It's funny to say you smoke because of the flavor or the taste, when, at the same time, smoking systematically destroys your ability to smoke. It kills your capability of experiencing the four basic taste buds we have, which is sweet, bitter, sour, and salty.

John R. Polito, in his book, *Freedom from Nicotine*, said it best: "you don't have taste buds in your lungs", wake up.

If you like the taste of chocolate or honey or other sweetener or other product, buy that product and enjoy it. You don't have to smoke cigs that have flavors; you are just adding more chemicals in the already huge amount of chemicals you are taking in already.

I remember I tried once menthol cigarettes. Oh, my God, I almost threw up and then returned to my tasteless, flavorless cigs. Why do you think I did that? You can give a smoker cigs that smell like poop and they will still smoke them! She smokes not for the flavor or the taste, she smokes because she is a drug addict. Nothing will stop her from getting her fix, to satisfy her urges, to prevent herself to be in a position where she will feel withdrawal symptoms.

Lesson Number 6: You smoke because you are addicted to nicotine and smoking tobacco cigarettes is the quickest, most efficient way to deliver nicotine directly into your brain. You don't smoke because you like the taste. Try and remember the first time you light a cigarette. Was that a pleasant experience? No, it wasn't. It was nasty and felt terrible.

Rationalization Number Seven: My coffee will never taste the same without smoking at the same time.

When I was 31, I was diagnosed with stomach and duodenum ulcer and smoking, except junk food and other factors, was responsible for my ulcer. My doctor told me to stop drinking and eating a lot of things. The first thing he said was to quit smoking because smoking destroys the inner layer of our stomach, the layer that protects us from our hydrochloric acid. By reducing this layer, the acid can create little wounds on the inside of my stomach, creating an ulcer. If not treated, a hole can be made, puncturing my stomach. From there, bleeding follows and unless you are lucky enough to get to the hospital in time so they can empty your stomach, cut you open, and seal the wound, you are dead before you can say, "One, two, three". The other thing he said I should stop was coffee. Caffeine has addictive properties like nicotine, but to a lesser degree. I told him that I can stop drinking coffee and other caffeinated drinks and sodas, but can't quit smoking. That's what I said to the doctor, that's what he heard from me that day.

Why am I telling you this story? Hmm, I don't know, maybe because I want you to see that you can live without coffee, and smoke, that this rationalization that coffee will never taste a good again without smoking is only in your thick head, like it was in my ignorant head ten years ago.

I did manage to stop drinking coffee but I did it gradually I reduced the number of cups I had per week until I got rid of the caffeine dependency but with caffeine, you can do that because it's not as addictive as nicotine. There are people who give themselves coffee enemas! Yes, they claim that they help the liver detoxify our body better and faster.

As I mentioned earlier, smoking dulls and reduces our ability to taste as we should. I remember it was 3 to 4 months after I stopped smoking and for about a week, I was in so much trouble. Everything started to taste better, stronger; I began to recognize flavors I never thought of. I felt so good again. My nose was having a party, I could smell odors dozens of feet away. Everything was so intense until my body found a way to control and acclimatize to my new found taste and smell.

Smoking kills your smell and taste abilities. When you smoke you don't smell and taste as good. Don't try to find an excuse like' but I sense that or feel that'. You don't, it's not reality that you smell or taste. It's a distorted reality, one that goes through the addictive filter of smoke and nicotine.

When you stop tobacco use and get your taste buds back, you will be able to enjoy your cup of morning coffee better; you be able to appreciate the flavor, taste, and aroma of a fresh ground coffee beans coffee.

Lesson Number 7: Stop smoking to get back your sense of smell and taste. What you taste and smell now is a bad copy of your suppressed senses brought upon you by the smoke and the toxins it contains. Stop smoking, free your mind, free your thoughts, and live life again as you should without the prison of nicotine.

Rationalization Number Eight: Smoking helps me focus and concentrate on the task ahead.

When I was a student, I never read or studied during the day if I had no morning classes the next day. I would read from 10 p.m. until 4 a.m. the next day and then go to sleep for about 8 hours, then wake up and attend the afternoon and night classes.

I never smoked when I was reading, or studying. I did drink a lot of coffee, mind you, I give you that. Smoking was a distraction for me and because my concentration was a concern because I would have to stop reading and smoke. I wasn't smoking all the time when I was reading, lost a lot of time from reading and also had to break my concentration every time I had to have a cigarette.

Now how on earth do you think smoking helps you focus? Yes, nicotine is a stimulant like caffeine. It raises your heartbeat by 17.5 times per minute, makes your blood pressure go up, it narrows your blood vessels, and creates hardening of the arteries, like meat and dairy do to your body. Another thing that completely contradicts the 'it helps me focus' rationalization is that massive quantities of carbon monoxide, one of the most deadly gases on this planet, is being pumped into your blood. In effect, this reduces the oxygen that can be carried by your bloodstream and results in lower oxygen to your brain .How is that helping you concentrate when your brain doesn't function 100%?

Also, nicotine, being a toxin, gradually kills your gray and white matter, which is important because you can't learn new stuff and focus without them.

Every two hours, which is the half-life of nicotine, you need to stop what you are doing, whether its work or whatever else, and get your dose, your fix. Regardless of what's going on around you, if you don't, you start shaking, and withdrawal symptoms start to appear .Oh, we don't want that to happen.

I realized, when researching this article and my book about smoking, that one of the reasons I was not eating breakfast or lunch was because I was a smoker. I mean, every time someone smokes, one of nicotine effects is to release fat and glucose into the blood from the liver, feeding me somehow. That's how smoking cuts your appetite.

By not eating right, though, and missing food, my blood sugar was always down and by smoking and releasing fat and glucose in my blood from the liver, as I said, it would give me a sense of fullness, making me not hungry anymore and thus being able to focus on my task.

I mean, think, when you are hungry, you want to eat to get that glucose into you and continue doing what you want to do. Instead of eating, I smoked, which had the same effect. Only, instead of getting the food from my mouth, my liver will supply it, making the hunger go away. The release of stored fat and glucose in my bloodstream enabled me to focus on the task ahead, making me think that it was smoking that helped me concentrate. Do you see the error of my actions here?

Lesson Number 8: Smoking doesn't assist you in focus or concentration .It does exactly the opposite. You need to break your concentration, break your focus, so you can smoke at least every two hours. You need to smoke to keep your nicotine blood serum levels to satisfying levels. It reduces the oxygen supply to your brain; I don't see how that will help you focus.

If you want to energize yourself and stimulate it naturally, go for a brisk walk for 10 minutes. Fresh, clean air and exercise are the best stimulants, and they do aid with your focus and concentration, not toxins like nicotine.

Rationalization Number Nine: I am smoking to kill boredom, otherwise, I don't

If you were not bored, then you wouldn't smoke. You think boredom makes you smoke so you can fill the void? Are you serious? You smoke because you are a drug addict, not because you are bored.

Let's analyze it a bit deeper. Yes, we are going to use our logic once again to prove to you how lame and stupid this rationalization is.

Why are we getting bored? Have you ever stop and thought, *Why do we get bored?* I tell you why. We get bored when we have nothing to do or at least our mind thinks we have nothing to do; there is always something to do. I rest by stopping what I am doing and do something else to change the focus. For example, if I get bored writing this article, then I will go downstairs and prepare food or do the dishes, or go outside and work on my garden. I make sure I don't have a dull minute in my life; I wasted 16 years smoking and being in this useless situation where the only thing that matters was to feed myself nicotine, which, by the way, is a natural insecticide! I used to inhale pesticide into my lungs, and I was under the impression I was doing something good for me, my friend, my companion, that it relieves my stress and helps me focus .Lies, all of them!

Boredom is a way that our brilliant body tells us to do something. Have you ever noticed that when you are bored, you have this edgy feeling that makes you get up off your butt and do something? That's our body's natural way of motivating us; it gives a bit of stress and anxiety so we will do something about our problem, our boredom, so it can reward us later with an excellent natural dopamine release as a bonus.

But guess what? Yes, you guessed right. Every time we get bored, we get a bit of stress, stress makes urine acidic, the body dumps nicotine from our bloodstream into our urine to make it more alkaline, and the smoker feels the withdrawal symptoms because of the rapid depletion of nicotine and lights a cigarette.

Nicotine saturates the brain's dopamine pathway receptors; a drug-induced dopamine dose is released at the same time nicotine stores up again, and the smoker thinks that smoking relieves boredom. In reality, you satisfied your addiction and, more importantly, missed the opportunity to do something amazing for yourself or for someone else .Instead of filling the void of boredom with something productive, you end up sitting on your butt, smoking cigarettes like a genuine drug addict and junkie you are.

I can't imagine all the things I could have done or accomplished with the time I wasted feeding my addiction. Instead, I could have learned how to play the guitar, something that was my passion as a kid. Wood sculpture, the list is endless, but I couldn't do them because every time I was bored, instead of using that time for something beneficial for me and my family, I just sat on my ass and smoked!

The other reason that smokers, and I, in the past, thought that smoking relieves boredom is that when you're bored, you have nothing to do so the things you do while in that state are more memorable when you usually smoke and do something else. One example is smoking and drinking coffee and talking with friends. Another is smoking while you are driving and listening to the radio. Get it? When you're bored, the actual movements of you taking a cigarette out of the package, putting it in your mouth, lighting it, taking a puff, and exhaling the smoke are the only thing that you are doing, thus you remember it better, giving you the impression that smoking relieves boredom.

Lesson Number 9: Smoking doesn't alleviate anything. It doesn't reduce stress, it doesn't relieve boredom either. Our nicotine addiction hijacks another natural way that the body has to makes us do something. By now, you should have seen the pattern. The truth is shaping, and you are starting to understand how this addiction works and how it is stealing your health and your life away from you gradually and methodically. Good news is that you can do something about it, you can stop right now and regain your freedom and your autonomy from a chemical called nicotine.

Rationalization Number Ten: After the divorce, I don't have much pleasure in my life. Smoking is one of them.

Hmm, pleasure and needs, wanting and genuine joy, what's the difference? Really, when you see your child taking its first steps, is that real joy and happiness that appears to your face from eyes to ear? Yes, I think it is.

When you've been working on a project at work for weeks now and it is finally finished, and it's fruitful and successful, then the pleasure and joy you feel are genuine.

Feeding yourself with a chemical that its primary function is to keep insects away from the tobacco plant is not joy, is not pleasure.

You think a heroin addict, when they prick themselves with needles to get their fix, to get their dose, is having feelings of pleasure or just satisfying a temporary addiction until the next fix and the next fix and the next fix?

How about someone snorting cocaine using his nostrils, you think that person is in pleasure? Is he happy, is he joyful? No, he is not, he is an addict. So are *you*, my friend. So I was eight years ago .I didn't smoke because it gave me pleasure, I satisfied my wanting, and that was it. There is a difference.

When you see a heroin addict on the side of the street coming towards you begging you for money, do you feel pity for them? Have you ever noticed or thought that maybe other people who don't smoke have the same feelings as you have for the heroin addict? Well ,let me tell you, they have them, I have them now for smokers. I see smokers and I pity them! As I am sure people did for me when I was a smoker. Something to keep in mind next time you decide to exclude yourself from the drug addict category when you see a heroin addict or cocaine addict whether in reality or the movies.

Saying that you feel pleasure when you smoke reminds me of the joke where a guy went to the doctor and told him, "Doc, whenever I use my right-hand index finger to touch something, it hurts!" and the doc says to him, "Don't poke with that finger, use your other index finger!"

It's the same thing, don't smoke, and find something else to do, something that will give you genuine pleasure and joy. Stop confusing addiction and the satisfaction of it with receiving pleasure in that cloudy mind of yours.

When you make love to your wife, fiancée, your partner ,you're giving and receiving pleasure. Pleasure is not a one-way street like smoking is. What does Nicotine give you? Nothing, you expect pleasure from a cigarette, but it gives you death.

Lesson Number 10: Things that give us genuine pleasure are the things, situation, and persons that are not killing us. Nicotine is taking your precious memories away; it deletes who you are from your brain, and the smoke with its 4,000 chemicals blackens your lungs and annihilates you methodically. The truth is that it's not pleasurable at all! Take action now, stop smoking, give it a try. You have nothing to lose, literally nothing to lose; you leave nothing behind, and you have everything to gain. Trust me, I know, I was you eight years ago. Come on, join me in a smoke-free nicotine life full of real and genuine pleasure and joy.

Rationalization Number Eleven: I don't know what people say, but I have the right to smoke, and it's my choice. I chose to smoke, no one makes me smoke.

I used to use that line, that it's my choice to smoke, that I am an adult, and I know what I am doing. I know that is not good for you but I will take that risk. A colleague of mine at work always tells me, "We are going to die anyway, at least I will die happy and get pleasure out of my life."

It's a powerful rationalization when a smoker tells you we are going to die anyway so why to stop smoking.

For years after I stopped smoking, I didn't have an argument to counteract this rationalization; it bothered me until one day, it clicked.

It's not how many years we are going to spend, it's the quality of year. We have a saying here in Cyprus, "few years but healthy years".

Well, when you smoke, all you can expect is indeed few years and hard, unhealthy years. Yes, of course, all of us will die at some point but why have a life filled with discomforts and diseases that are caused by the direct or indirect actions of smoking?

I don't think any smoker today would like to be at the receiving end of a table where a man or a woman in a white robe will tell him or her that they have terminal lung cancer, esophageal cancer, or any other kind of cancer.

I don't think any smoker today would like to hear that they have emphysema and so on.

When the withdrawal symptoms start to kick in, because you didn't have the chance to satisfy your addiction in that exact moment, choosing to smoke or not to smoke is the only *real* choice you make when you are a smoker and a nicotine addict. All the other actions are not your choice.

From the first puff you took, you gave away your ability to choose things as far as smoking is concerned.

If you had a choice, you will never continue buying them, smoking them, and you would have stopped. You are a drug addict like I was a year ago, and you lost your autonomy and free will to a drug called nicotine.

Smoking is not a choice I said it before, and I say it again, it's a very effective way of delivering a highly toxic and addictive chemical into your brain and body.

People who say they don't care what happens to them because of their smoking have some emotional and psychological issues that they need to resolve.

A healthy mind doesn't want to kill itself; a healthy mind wants to occupy its time with activities that promote a healthy status of life.

A healthy life doesn't commit suicide (slowly, I'll give you that) by smoking. That's what I was doing when I was a smoker. I had issues, I was depressed, and I had emotional insecurities and psychological fear. I was escaping all of these things by smoking, by drugging myself to forget. It's the same thing an alcoholic does, to forget about their problems, they drown themselves in booze. Instead of facing my problems, I was escaping to a false nirvana that everything was fine with me, that it was my choice to smoke. I don't think so; I know that now.

Lesson Number 11: Smoking is not a choice, a choice is to get up in the morning and make breakfast for your love ones. A choice is to start going to the gym, so you be a healthier person, a choice is to stop smoking get rid of nicotine and have a healthier, more meaningful life, on an emotional, psychological, and physiological level. Saying your addiction a choice is like an alcoholic saying I chose to drink wine. Do you get it? Others have an addiction to heroin, cocaine, meth, alcohol, yours is nicotine, like it was for me eight years ago, but I chose to get rid of it, that's the only genuine real choice you have.

Rationalization Number Twelve: It's a habit, nothing to worry about, I can stop whenever I want.

This rationalization is probably the most common one in smokers' heads, it's a habit, it's just a nasty habit, and it's a bad habit. Society doesn't make it any easier to see the truth. Not too many years ago, we had commercials on TV, advertising cigs. I remember when I was little, I would watch this commercial with this cowboy, the Marlboro man. A macho man smoking, boy, I got the wrong messages, but my words were closer to home, my father, who I adore, also smoked .I hated that about him when I was growing up, but later, I ended up like him, a smoker. Talking about subliminal messages.

Society is not hard enough on smokers because nicotine is still legal and I say still legal because I dream of the day where nicotine will be illegal like all the drugs, like heroin, cocaine, and others.

Also, society likes to use soft language when it comes to concepts or real situations where they have trouble facing the truth. Society has real trouble when meeting with reality, so we use soft language .Let me give you an example. In the World War I, people who couldn't handle the inhuman conditions of war had either two choices: take care of it or snap. That state where our nervous system cannot process any more information or can't manage existing information was called Shell shock. It was honest and direct, and it shows the real situation of the people who have it. Over the years, and with every new war and with every new generation, the same condition managed to transform itself from Shell Shock to Battle Fatigue, to Operational Exhaustion to Post Traumatic Stress Disorder, hiding the truth about the situation altogether and making us the rest of feel better.

Well, it's the same with smoking. The fact is, it's a dangerous and dirty (smoke, fire, tar) mechanism that its sole purpose is to deliver a highly addictive and hazardous toxin into our heads and bodies. But for non-smokers and smokers, it sounds better to hide the truth and makes us feel better if we christen it a nasty little habit. Well, it is disgusting, I give you that, but it's not little. Every year, 5 million people on this planet die from smoking-related illnesses. And, it's not a habit, it's a deadly addiction.

You can see people smoke in the movies, in the street, everywhere. No wonder everyone thinks is an evil, nasty habit. Well, it's not a habit. It's an addiction and presenting it as a habit is wrong as it has a direct negative effect on the youth. Kids and teenagers looking at smoking as a habit and not as a deadly addiction will experiment, and it only takes one puff to get hooked as Joel Spitzer shows in his book, *Not Another Puff*(put a link to the book here),a man who knows more about smoking and how to quit than everyone else combined on this planet.

If I want to make a habit, exercising some yoga in the morning before I go to work for 10 to 15 minutes, I will need to apply myself and repeat those exercises for at least a month for it to become a habit, something that my body will ask for. And the reverse, if you want to stop a habit, you need to stop doing it for at least 3 to 4 weeks and then your body will stop asking for it.

The irony was that I had this notion in my head that if I managed to quit smoking for three weeks, then I will not start again. It worked for me, I went with wrong thinking but ended up with positive results. Seven years ago, when I did my final and successful attempt to stop smoking, I wish I knew that it only takes three days to get rid of nicotine from my system. I would have educated myself better on how to respond to the social situations where I used to smoke, then I am sure I would have quit easier without as many withdrawal symptoms and false fears.

When someone takes a puff, that's it, they instantly becomes an addict until they stop smoking. They don't have to smoke cigarettes continuously for a month to become an addict, you are from the first puff. That's it, that's the secret of how tobacco companies hook you up.

It's not a habit, it's an addiction, and if you admit it, you will have greater chances of stopping and not considering it a habit like I did.

Lesson Number 12: A pattern needs time to become something that you will do every day, and from all the experience I have, and the books I read, it takes 3 to 4 weeks or repeated application. Smoking doesn't need that kind of use. With your first puff of smoke, you are officially a drug addict. Make the distinction between habitual actions, like going to the gym every day, or writing 1,000 words every day, and activities you do because you are afraid of the withdrawal symptoms of nicotine depletion. You are smarter than this; you now know that smoking is not a habit but rather, a very efficient delivery mechanism of nicotine, a toxic and highly addictive drug.

Rationalization Number Thirteen: If I quit smoking, I will lose all of my friends.

This rationalization was always on my mind. In the back of my sick, addicted mind, I had this notion that because of the smoking, I was more sociable, I was friendlier somehow, that because of my smoking "habit", I was making new friends. The reality of the matter was far, far away from my way of distorted thinking under the nicotine addiction.

The only "friends" I had were other smokers and a few people who tolerated me.

Let me ask you this, what do you think a beautiful, non-smoking woman and a handsome non-smoking man would prefer?

A.   A smoker who, every time he or she speaks to you, you feel like you put your mouth over the exhaust of a car. She or he smells smoke all the time even when they don't smoke. They will not be able to have a conversation or going traveling because now and then, he or she must stop whatever you are doing so he or she will smoke. Yellow fingers and teeth. They cannot enjoy a coffee together because the smoker wants to smoke, with the result being all that smoke coming your way, making you a secondary or a passive smoker. They will not be able to go out to a restaurant because the smoker will want to sit where he or she can smoke, which drowns you in carcinogens. Also, they will worry about your health, even if you don't, adding more stress and anxiety to their already busy life. They will not be able to do athletics together because let's face it, you will die on the first 5 meters of vigorous exercise. Parents who smoke increases the chances of having kids with respiratory problems and other health issues.

B.   A non-smoker, who doesn't have the breath of a chimney, doesn't stink of smoke, and has beautiful white teeth and clean fingers.

Who actually can enjoy a cup of coffee and can see you because the fog of smoke that was coming from the smokers' mouth is not there, enjoy a nice, lovely, smoke-free lunch in a restaurant. Can raise a healthy family together, not leaving them to worry that you might drop dead any moment from lung cancer, who can enjoy athletics and sports with you.

Which of the two people I just described have more opportunities to meet and make friends? A smoker or a non-smoker? The answer, of course, is so obvious that I am so angry that I had to describe the categories in the first place. The non-smoker, the non-heroin addict, the non-cocaine addict, the non-meth addict of course!

Wake up, why on earth would I want to be with a person who has no regard for their personal health and sometimes hygiene and doesn't care about mine either? I want to be with people who care about me, who love me and want to be my friend, not people who are trying to kill me every time they exhale a cloud of carcinogens towards me, gassing me!

A big percentage of smokers want to stop smoking. They want to quit; they realized they are trapped into a situation that in their eyes cannot escape. Wouldn't it be wonderful if they had a friend who succeeded in quitting and wouldn't it be amazing if you could show them the way and help them stop, too?

Smokers have fears, lots of them. God, I know I had a zillion when I was under the influence of nicotine. Some are real, but most of them are in their heads. They are psychological fears, they are not real at all. All you need to do is think of something else, and the fear will go away.

Quitting smoking and fearing that you will lose your friends. It is a psychological fear, it's not real. Years of smoking and talking with your buddies, smoking and drinking coffee or other beverages with your friends, smoking and doing anything with your friends has created a sick association that if you quit, then you will lose your friends, too. You fear that everything else you were doing and smoking at the same time will end because you as an addict smoked in every aspect of your life. That's why when many smokers decide to stop tobacco use, a month from now, and they are still fine with it, they are cool; they say, "I have time to smoke a few more cigarettes." The two weeks mark comes, and they are still okay, but they start to feel a bit pressured that they might give up smoking. Give up is another nice phrase smokers use to provide some value to their worthless addiction. The big day comes that they need to go down to a clinic or a cessation center, and they freeze, they stay home, they are so afraid that if they stop smoking, their life will change for the worse somehow. They will lose their friends, lose everything they have been doing while smoking at the same time. Coffee, eating, sex, everything. They think that by stopping smoking their lives will be over!

Isn't that just crazy? Well, for us non-smokers, it is, but for an addict, it is not. You need to realize something, that your life is ending little by little every time you light a cig and take that puff; you are losing friends while you smoke and not the other way around.

Lesson Number 13: Smoking alienates you and makes you antisocial, it keeps you away from people who care about you and want what is best for you. By quitting smoking, you will be able to make more friends than before, enjoy life's social advantages to the fullest and your life will *begin*, not *end* like you thought it would. Trust me when I say this, after two months of no smoking, a new and exciting world of senses, opportunities, and capabilities opened up to me that I was so high on life, I knew I never wanted to use a drug to get *high* again in my life. Also, on a final note, if you quit, you will see from your already existing "friends", who has friendship feelings towards you, and you be able to find out your real and genuine friends. Worth a shot!

Rationalization Number Fourteen: I can't stop, I really can't! I tried so many times, I am going to face the fact that I will die a smoker.

You can do whatever you want; you need to relax and, no, I don't mean light a cigarette. Just take deep breaths and fuel that beautiful mind of yours with pure oxygen, not carbon monoxide.

Just sit on your couch or a chair anywhere that you feel comfortable. Take a deep breath through your nose, hold it, count to5, and then exhale through your mouth.

You will probably get a little bit dizzy because you gave your brain more oxygen than it is accustomed to with your smoking and all.

Do this exercise as many times as you need achieve complete relaxation.

When you reach that point, and you will understand when you arrive at that point, because you will feel nothing, you will be in an essential emptiness; your mind is empty of the worries, problems, and fears of everyday life.

At that point, I want you to remember the life you had as a non-smoker and I want you to remember the feeling of autonomy and independence you had.

Remember that you had a life without smoking, and you were just fine.

Do that every time you think you are not able to quit; I guarantee you, it will change your mind.

When I was a little boy, my beloved mother would always say to me, when I was sad or down, "There is no 'I can't', there is only 'I won't'."

You are telling me that you are afraid of a chemical like nicotine, which leaves your body in the first three days after you stop smoking? Yes, it's addictive, duh, but are you telling me you are so weak that you can't physically stop putting those tubes of cancer in your mouth?

You are not *weak*, okay? Just quit smoking. You will have withdrawal symptoms; of course, you will. You had a poison dictate your life for I don't know how many years. My magic number was 16 years, I was killing myself for 16 years and for what? What? Nothing, smoking offered me nothing, zilch. It only alienated me from people I might had become good friends with, even maybe missed the opportunity to meet the woman of my life, because of stupid smoking.

I was killing myself day in and day out. With every single puff, I was putting my health and the health the people around me, loved ones or strangers, in danger.

After three days, you have no *physiological* addiction, you have nothing to keep you back. You have no excuse to smoke again because the addiction is out of your system; that's how easy it is.

You need to do the hard work. For me, I learned a long time ago, and the hard way, that there is no *easy* or *difficult* tasks in life. There is being lazy and sitting on your butt, doing nothing, and getting off that couch and learning, practicing, experimenting ,and becoming knowledgeable .Stop being an *ignorant* junkie and use the knowledge you learned from this article and *do* something!

Quitting smoking for me .As I see it now that I have been smoking and nicotine free for seven years now, it is 1% nicotine addiction (in 72 hours, it's out of your system after you quit) and 99% psychological fear. Guess what, though, irrational concerns are not *real*, they are in your head, they are like these rationalizations I already mentioned and the ones after this.

When you stop smoking, your life will not be *over*. It will *start!* You will not lose friends, you will *gain* even more friends. You will be able to be social, play with your kids more, travel more, satisfy that woman of yours more (wink), or for the ladies, please your man even more (wink again). You can do sports, you can use that hour you wasted on smoking to do *something else*. Learn how to play an instrument, start running, swimming, walking, or start doing hobbies you always said you *don't have time for*. Well, guess what? When you stop smoking, you will. Think of all the money you save, all the trips you can do, the things you can buy for you and your family and your friends!

Stop being afraid. It's this simple, let me repeat it for you.

You stop smoking. After 72 hours, nicotine, that "bitch", a big percentage of it is out of your system, then you need to deal with the psychological fear, and there are not that many. Trust me, you are not going to have nightmares or demons hunting you down. You need to deal with the fact that you need to drink coffee, without smoking. Try it, it might taste and smell better because you stop smoking ;the same thing with food.

Holidays are coming, you used to smoke during them, right? Well, train yourself not to smoke, prepare yourself when the psychological fear comes. I repeat, after 72 hours, you will not have any physiological urges; it's in your head. I wish I knew that when I stopped smoking, I could have had a smoother, easier time quitting.

Take a piece of paper and program as best as you can what you will do when you feel like smoking after the 72 hours, when you have no reason physiologically to smoke, and find alternatives.

I give you a practical example of what I did when I had smoking desires.

I had toothpicks with me. I also cut plastic straws in small pieces. I had snacks with me and also a chair that I had in the room, and I named that the airplane chair. I tell you what I mean by that.

When the desire struck, I would chew on the straws, I would eat and drink, yes, eat junk food; it's more important to associate everything you did with smoking than thinking if you gain a few pounds now, you can deal with the pounds later. De-program yourself with the mechanical act of smoking and doing everyday things you need to break this weak association.

And finally, if the desire was very strong, I would go and sit on the airplane chair, and pretend I was on a trip to the Bahamas. D oyou know what is not allowed on the plane? SMOKING, it helped me, the airplane chair.

Another thing I would do was the car seat, but I had my nephew in the back. I would pretend I was driving my sweet nephews to play ball together at the park. Guess what desire was gone? The desire to smoke.

Do your homework, program and re-teach yourself to live without a cigarette. Is it going to be easy? That's the whole point, there is no easy or difficult. Stop using these words, there is you did your homework and invested the time, or you didn't.

Lesson Number 14: When there is a will, there is a way, and I just showed it you. What are you going to do with it? It's your choice!

Rationalization Number Fifteen: Why quit? I am fine, I still have my health.

Exactly, you drug addicted, ignorant person, like the one I was eight years ago, and I was counting on my good immune system. I was counting on my good physical condition, I was relying on my youth to convince myself that smoking was okay and that nothing will happen to me. I am lucky, I am not like the others, bad things happen to other people, not me, I am special!

What a load of *crap ,*excuse my French here, but it is.

It's sad that people, and I, I am not excluding myself, have to suffer to learn. I mean, if I didn't have the stomach ulcer and the doctor never told me to quit smoking, I would never have related the fact that smoking sends more people to their grave than all the illegal drugs together! Think about that.

What was wrong with me? Oh, wait, I was a drug addict! I am happy, yes, glad that I got that stomach ulcer. It made me think, it forced me to reevaluate my actions, it forced me to see that I am not invincible like I thought I was. We are not immortals, people. Wake up, that's only in the movies, we are not Connor MacLeod from the famous movie "Highlander", and even Connor Macleod wasn't smoking. Think about that!

Yes, you are still healthy. Still is the word, why take the chance, why? I mean, I am scared to shit every time I do my annual exams, blood, and others to see if I have a cancer cell in my body. Every year, I thank myself that I stopped smoking and until I reach 15 years of non-smoking, where you come to the health status of a non-smoker, I will worry.

I don't know what 16 years of smoking did to my body. I don't, but you know what? I am glad that I quit. I am me now. I have control of my actions, I am not pushed around by a chemical like nicotine.

I run marathons now as a hobby. I mean if a fat, nicotine addict like me managed to be smoke and nicotine free and run marathons for a hobby, everything is possible.

When the world health organization says smoking kills, they are not just saying it for kicks .It kills.

When an earthquake hits and levels an entire city, it doesn't give any warnings. It just hits. Same thing with smoking. When it hits, you will realize at that precise moment how stupid and ignorant you were. You will wish you never smoked. The funny thing is that you could go cold turkey right now when you heard, for example, that you have emphysema, lung cancer, or another nasty smoking related illness and disease. Why do you have to suffer to quit and even if you quit, it will mean nothing because you are going to be dead anyway?

Lesson Number 15: Stop now before it's too late. It's never too late, take your life back, do not be arrogant and conceited. Do not end up like the famous actor, Yul Bryner, who ,in his last interview, said that the only thing he regretted doing was smoking and he was urging people not to. Don't be Yul Brenner as far as smoking is concerned. Live, stop smoking now.

Rationalization Number Sixteen: It's hard to quit. I am always confronted by monsters and demons, I can't escape them.

I am going to be easy on you with this rationalization because I've been there and I know what it means to smokers when they say, "I can't quit because I am afraid of the unknown", but instead of using the word 'unknown', they use something that is closer to home, 'demons and monsters'.

Only ignorant people believe in monsters and demons. It's as plain as that. I think all the arguments I presented here debunking the previous rationalizations are enough to see that there are no monsters and daemons out there to get you after you quit smoking. There is only you and how much you are willing to work not to take another puff in your life, like Joel Spitzer always says and always finishes his videos in YouTube and in his book Never take another puff.

When I was 7 or 8, I don't remember, we used to live in my aunt's house because, well, we didn't have a house of our own. It took years for father to build it on his own. Me and my brother, we would never go to bed unless there was this doll head positioned above a lamp which was on the wall across our beds. That doll head was our guardian, she protected us from the monsters that lived in the dark.

Were our fears real? What do you think? Of course not. It was in our heads. There are no monsters living in the dark. It's night and then day comes, and then night again, and soon. That happens because the earth revolves around her axis and around the sun!

There are no demons or monsters or any other fears after you quit smoking. There is willingness to work on ridding yourself of a deadly addiction and also educate yourself to become a new version of you, a version who doesn't need to kill him/herself anymore or anyone around you.

Nicotine is just a chemical and it's really strong, I'll grant you that, but you are a complex human being capable of making trillions of decisions in a fraction of a second. You are much much smarter than a chemical; you don't have to be stronger to win this war between you and your drug, you need to be smarter!

Lesson Number 16: I hope you did learn your lesson after reading this article. I have nothing else to add at the moment, I only hope I will see you on the other side, my friend. Have a healthy and happy day.

My Warmest Regards,

Andreas Michaelides

Sources that will help you quit smoking:

I will give you three names, you don't need anything else and you are half way there to a smoke free, nicotine free life. Enjoy!

Joel   Spizer   -
http://www.joelspitzer.com/mystory.htm

Book, *NeverTake Another Puff* –http://whyquit.com/joel/ntap.pdf completely free to download.

YouTube channel https://www.youtube.com/user/joelspitz

Quit Smoking Library http://whyquit.com/joel/

John R. Polito - http://whyquit.com/JohnBio.html

YouTube channel https://www.youtube.com/user/JohnRPolito

Book, *Freedom from Nicotine – A Journey Home* - http://whyquit.com/ffn/– completely free to download.

Allen Carr–Died from Lung Cancer on November 29, 2006, at age 72. God rest his soul.

Webpage http://www.allencarr.com/

YouTube   videos–
https://www.youtube.com/watch?v=xRHc1XKId6A&list=PL_O
e4cHGpavNZK3icPVQjoXCjfdXD9DAS

There are 199 of them!

Other books by Andreas Michaelides

Thirsty For Health

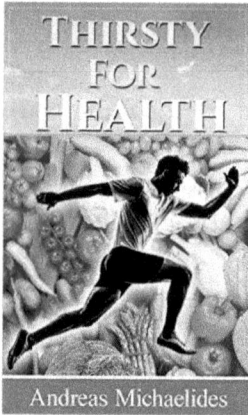

A truly eye opening book that should and will make your question yourself and everything you have done so far diet and lifestyle wise. Obesity, caffeine and junk food addiction, smoking and digestive problems? This is the place you can start answering your most asked questions. A book you wish you had found earlier, an amazing story that had to be told in order to help others not to go through the same misery. In these pages you will learn how to regain control over your life, how to find strength from within in order to go through life's numerous challenges, successfully overcome addictions and finally tune in to genuine health and happiness. You are the alchemist, the architect of your life and no one else but you have the power to make the change. Be the change that you want to see in the world. You can start now and this book will help you do that and more and you will also learn how to live long and live well.

The Food I Grew Up With...Veganized!

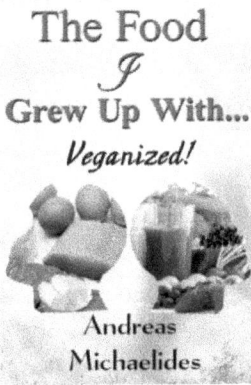

The Food
I
Grew Up With...
Veganized!

Andreas
Michaelides

I wrote this book first to thank my mother for never letting me without food on the table and secondly to show to people out there that they can thrive on a plant based diet and the most important of all they don't have to start from zero as food is concerned I hope I will show with this book that you can transform many of your old food into new versions of plant based ones. This book is not a cookbook although it contains a lot of the food recipes I used to and still eating today. All the recipes are a result of many interviews with my mother which without her this book would never be possible. This book basically shows one aspect of my psyche as food is concerned and how I deal with it transitioning from an omnivore to a herbivore.

How to train and finish your first 5k race.

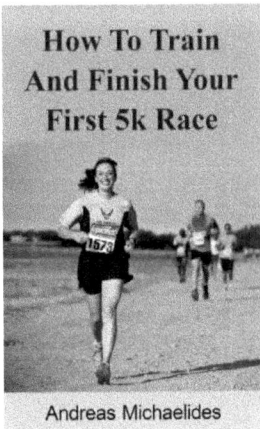

How To Train
And Finish Your
First 5k Race

Andreas Michaelides

You can watch other people running on the TV, playing football, basketball, or baseball. At least those guys are getting paid to run and jump and tackle. Why should you go through this torture of actually getting up from your soft chair and making yourself go through this ordeal? Why would you enter this nightmare? Why not continue your ignorant bliss of a lovely sedentary life where all you need to do is push the buttons of a remote control and then people in the box can live your desires, your fantasies, your dreams, and ultimately, your life?

My weight loss journey: How I lost 44 pounds and never gained them back using a plant based diet

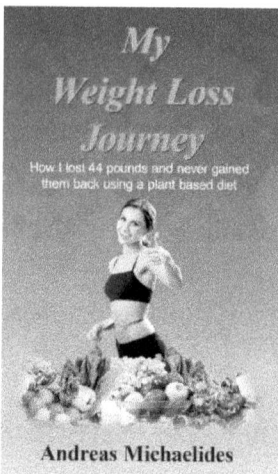

My
Weight Loss
Journey

How I lost 44 pounds and never gained them back using a plant based diet

Andreas Michaelides

Although I never expected to drag myself out of the house and go for a run, after I finished those first three rounds at the high school track in my village, everything changed. I was so exhausted—which was an indicator of how lacking my physical fitness was—but after all the discomfort, itching, and rash in various places due to friction from excess fat, for the first time, I felt renewed, and memories of running and coming in first place in high school reminded me of how I used to be compared to how I was after those three laps around the track.

It made my eyes water; I was alone in the middle of the track under an April sky full of stars when tears of mixed feelings started pouring down from my eyes. Emotionally and psychologically, it was a turning point for me, and it also made me even more determined to become that lean, mean running machine I used to be. It was right there in that single moment that I saw the path I had to follow.

Please write a review.

REVIEW
REVIEW
REVIEW

I consider myself as a person that wants to think that I am constantly improving my books, my work and myself. I am always trying to deliver to my readers the best quality and current information out there as my area of interest and expertise is concern which is Health, Nutrition and Exercise.

In order to accomplish that I need feedback from you and the only feedback I know that will help me achieve a relative perfection in all areas of my life is your valuable reviews so I know where I am wrong or where I have made mistakes and errors.

There is no such thing as a perfect book out there, perfection for one person is a sloppy work for other, so in order to satisfy as much as people out there my books need to be updated regularly and it doesn't matter if it is in electronic form (kindle) or paperback form.

If you found this book useful, please leave your review with all your thoughts, don't hold back, it will only take a few minutes of your time.

If you didn't like this book, please let me know by contacting me and I will give my best shot to fix the issue.

Thank you very much,

My warmest regards

Andreas Michaelides

www.ingramcontent.com/pod-product-compliance
Lightning Source LLC
Chambersburg PA
CBHW071032280326
41935CB00011B/1541